BUILD A HEALTHY LIVING YOU CAN BE PROUD OF

7 EASY STEPS TO SUCCESS

BY

NEYFI DEL ROSARIO

COPYRIGHT

ABOUT ME

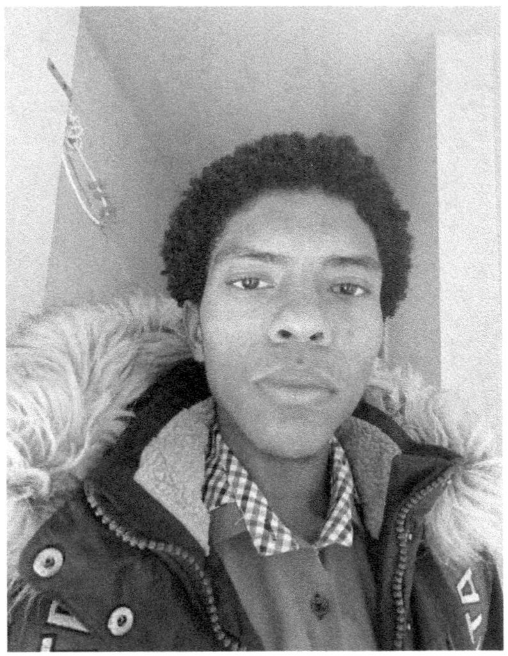

My name is Neyfi Del Rosario and I am an athlete. I am learning as much as I can and discovering my purpose in life, that changed my outlook in life forever. I will continue to learn and become better, smarter, stronger, and more knowledgeable. I want to take you with me through my journey to become the best and better version of myself. With your help, I will be able to love and enjoy life by inspiring others to be as successful in their health journey, and seek purpose.

DEDICATION

This book is for you. The reader.

CHAPTER I

QUALITY MATTERS

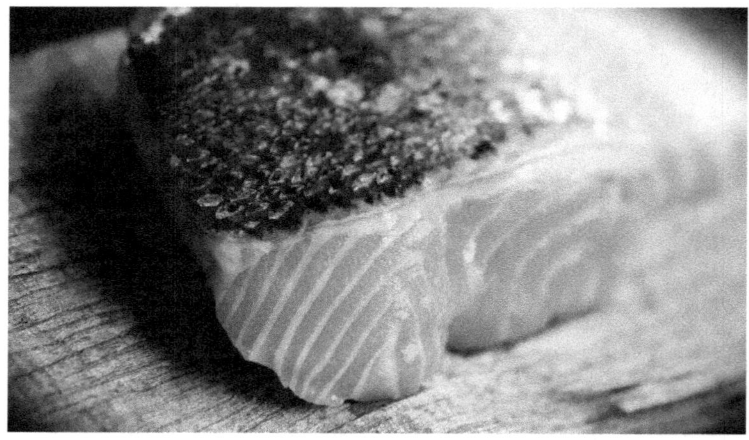

Being able to build a healthy lifestyle is a great achievement. To be able to be proud of your lifestyle if they are a couple of rules that you need to keep in mind. There are things that will help you achieve success and to become the best person that you can be. In this book, I will be teaching you easy and simple steps to remember and they will make your healthy lifestyle easier. You will be able to live a healthy lifestyle without stressing yourself about it. You will learn about the support of others and how you can help others while achieving a healthy lifestyle. You learn how goals in your life can be so helpful. You will learn how to enjoy a healthy lifestyle. This book will give you my simple eight steps that helped me find a healthy lifestyle. I will give you all my tips and secrets about a healthy lifestyle.

The first thing I always tell people to keep in mind is the most important thing. In a healthy lifestyle, you need quality. You need to look for quality as much as you can. By quality I mean you need to buy the best quality foods that you can afford. Having a better quality of food is an amazing opportunity that can guide you to a better lifestyle. The first step in quality is to look for the least processed foods you can find. Looking for minimally processed foods can be difficult at times. Look for foods that were not modified by human Beings. Non processed foods have better health benefits than buying processed food. Whole Foods like broccoli, salmon, and spinach have many health benefits. These benefits will be described throughout this book.

    To take this first step you need to focus on the quality of the food that you're buying. The first step is to check if they come in a box or not. It is very likely that many processed foods like pasta, bread, and prepackaged food are not the healthiest choices you can make. These processed foods are made in a factory. This allows many manufacturers to add ingredients that are not naturally found in foods. Many of these ingredients can be very harmful to your health. To know which ingredients are good or bad you need to check the labels. Check on the label if they have chemicals or not. If you do not know how to say the chemical or you do not have these chemicals in your kitchen you should not buy it. It is better not to take the chance on chemicals that may be harmful to you. It's better to limit the number of processed foods that you buy. Many processed foods can include things like frozen foods, pre-made foods, prepackaged meals, and processed meats. These man-made foods are very convenient for you. This allows more people to buy them because they are easier to consume. Sometimes the easiest and most abundant route is not the best route. Most of the time we have to take the harder route to make a better for ourselves.

You might be wondering, how can eating quality foods help me? This is simple: buying more wholesome foods can lead to a greater intake of nutrients and minerals that you need throughout your day. Many of these foods that are wholesome foods can lead to a reduction in type 2 diabetes, reductions of cancer, and reduction of inflammation. Later in this book, I point out and explain these health benefits.

I ask that you have better quality foods so it can lead you to not only a better healthy lifestyle but also in the relationships and quality of life that you have. By starting to look for quality foods, will lead you to look for quality everywhere. You will not be paying extra for the brands or buying something because someone else buys it. You start looking for quality instead of quantity or brand. You will learn a skill that will carry over to other aspects of your life. You learned what quality means to you and what quality does to your health. The people that you surround yourself with represent quality, the type of job that you do will show quality, and the quality of exercise that you do for your body will be quality. Quality is vital to have a healthy living. Always look for the best quality that you can afford. For example, if I can afford grass-fed organic beef, I will not buy grain-fed beef. My reason is grass-fed beef has more omega-3 fatty acids than omega-6 fatty acids. This is important because omega-3 fatty acids will reduce inflammation in my body. Later in this book, you will learn about how to balance your omega-3 and omega-6 fatty acids. You will learn about the effect of inflammation and the creation of tissues in your body.

Quality also translates to the type of supplementation that you get in your daily life. You need to know where to get good supplementation and which are the foods that contain the right amount of nutrients for you. You will know how to have a wholesome healthy diet that will allow you to increase your longevity and quality of life. There are many minerals and vitamins like sodium, potassium, omega-3 fatty acids, and vitamin D. These are minerals and vitamins that the majority of society is deficient in. This deficiency is caused by poor health habits and low-quality foods. Later in this book, you will learn what foods and supplements you can take to balance your healthy lifestyle. This can potentially lead you to have a longer, better, and quality life.

Exercise can lead you to a better and healthier lifestyle. I will tell you which are the exercises that I did and still do to become the better version that I am today. These exercises can be anything that you enjoy doing and can allow you to move your body in a way that you enjoy it. Exercise will make you feel great and accomplished by finishing a workout. You will learn how walking, running, and aerobic exercise can be a great way to start your healthy journey to success. There are many small things that will allow you to achieve and create a lifestyle that you can be proud of. You will learn about the exercises that I do to reduce stress and why it's important to lower stress as much as possible.

The most important part of a healthy lifestyle is to have a goal. A quality life cannot be started if you do not know where to go or what you want. This book will teach you three easy steps for you to follow and achieve many successful goals. This will allow you to have the motivation and direction of where you want to be and where you want to go. I will be teaching you about my mistakes and the things you should avoid to find a healthier, longer, and quality life.

Quality is a way for you to determine success. Think about quality as a business, if you're a business owner, and you decide that you sell your services for a cheaper price to attract more clients. This will end up devaluing your business. You will attract more customers but the type of customers will be a cheaper, lower-quality customer. Your quality of lifestyle works the same way. If you decide to buy because of convenience or buy because of quantity, you will end up with a cheaper type of life. Furthermore, the type of people that you surround yourself with can determine the type of quality healthy life you can have. For example, if you have a friend that you see on a regular basis. every single time you see this friend you two will eat unhealthy foods every single time you see each other. This can potentially lower the type of quality life that you have. The steps that I would take in this situation is to tell the person that you are looking for a better quality of life and you cannot eat those foods anymore. If this person is a high-quality person they will understand and respect your decision of having a better quality life. You will inspire others around you to start their journey to a better quality of life themselves. You will improve your life so much that other people would love to join you and support you to have a better quality of life.

A healthy living that you can be proud of. This means having a quality life that can have many motivational moments and teaching moments in your life. For example, You need a goal, Goals need to be specific. Your goal should say what you want, the things you'll do to get it, how long you want to do it for, and why. You should repeat this goal to yourself every morning and every night. This will lead you to go from thinking that your goal is impossible, to believe in your goal, to yourself becoming the thing that you believe. I always use myself as an example, when I was 11 years old, I started playing guitar. My goal was to become as good as a Rockstar. I used to play about 2 hours every single day to become better. I said "I want to be better" so much that I believed I could become better. Today, I might not be the best guitarist in the world but I can assure you I can not only play blindfolded behind my head. But I can take a guitar apart, fix it to the best of my abilities, and give it to someone that will be happy because their guitar works again.

Having quality goals can lead you to success. All you need to do is repeat your goal as much as you can. You will start believing and you will become what you believe. Later in this book, you will learn my step by step process to create your ultimate goal. These steps will not only help you in a healthy lifestyle you can be proud of but also help you in other aspects of your life. They can help you in your career and your ideas. After reading this book, you will have high-quality information that you will be able to research and teach others about the wonders of being healthy. Having a quality life will lead you to tell others about the thing that you do to become healthy. Being able to spread quality information with other people will lead to a healthy revolution in today's society. You need to seek quality as much as you can in every aspect of your life. It is not enough to conform with "good enough." You need to look for a quality lifestyle that will allow you to strive for greatness and success. Everything that you do this would have to be the best quality of service that you can give, the best quality of work you can do, and the best quality of foods that you can eat.

This simple change can lead you to a healthier, longer, and better quality of life by itself. I do not want you to stop there, I want you to seek for quality in your daily work daily life. Look for quality in every relationship you make. A relationship should be an opportunity to grow with someone, an opportunity for you to grow if the opportunity to grow is not there anymore, the relationship is done and it's time to move on. Look for quality people that will allow you more quality in your life. There are people that will help you achieve and grow your goals with you. The point of having a healthy lifestyle it's not only about the food you eat, but it's also not only about losing weight. It's also about your relationships and actions that you take on your daily life. There's no point in eating healthy food and having a stressful relationship. That will only lead you to have high stress that will counteract the good benefits of a healthy diet. There's no point in looking for quality on exercises if the food you eat will not provide the quality that you need. Look to be the best person that you can be. Allowing yourself to grow and look for the small things in life that will allow you to find quality. Find things that will help you achieve your goals. This will make you have a healthy living you can be proud of. Myself at the beginning of my healthy living I was surrounded by people who told me all the time "you will not make it." I knew I had to do something about my health and lifestyle that I was living in. The first step that I took was to look for people that have the same mentality as me. This allowed me to grow on all goals and the things that I wanted to accomplish. Even if many of my goals sound impossible. Having Good quality people in my life allows me to achieve my goals and be able to seek for quality in every moment of my life. I am not only looking for healthy choices in the supermarket, but I'm also looking for healthy choices about my life, success, and the people that I surround myself with. My second biggest change I did was looking for the best quality of food that I could afford. I stopped eating from fast-food restaurants, I stopped eating unhealthy foods. Foods like pizza and ice cream. I stopped thinking about convenience and started thinking about my future. I vision myself being healthy in my nineties. I want to live a long healthy life that is of high quality. I want to be able to spread quality to other people and create a healthy community. I want to create a health revolution that today's society needs. If I made a change in my lifestyle from eating habits to new relationships and important knowledge about goals, you can also change your life and you can become a better you.

CHAPTER II

THINGS TO AVOID

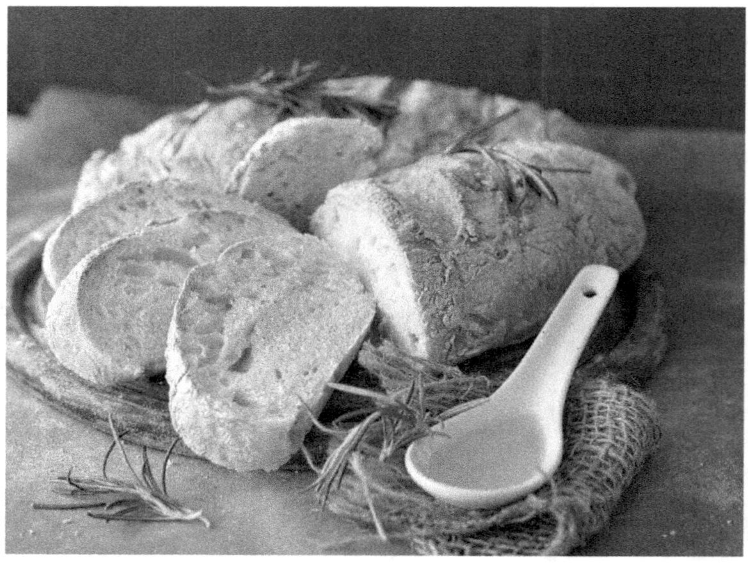

In a healthy lifestyle, the first thing we have to think about is the type of food that we're eating. Many people do not think about the type of food they eat makes a huge difference in their health. Many of these people believe that most health issues come from inherited genetic code they got from their parents. These people are not wrong. There are people who are more predisposed to be affected by diseases than other people. Many of these problems can be avoided by adjusting your diet to a healthy diet. There are many foods you need to avoid to have the healthiest diet that you can have. I am a believer in low carbs and ketogenic diets. The absence of carbohydrates and processed foods that are taken into consideration while following these diets are one of the reasons that many diseases can be avoided or reversed.

Highly processed foods and carbohydrates must be avoided to have a healthy lifestyle. Carbohydrates are everywhere. They are the most abundant source of energy of food in the world. Carbohydrates are metabolized in the body in the first second they enter your mouth. You have special enzymes in your mouth that specialize in breaking down the long starch chains of carbs many foods have. Foods like bread, potato, and cookies are made up of many long chains of starches. By the time these carbohydrates reach your stomach, they are in the simplest form of sugar, glucose. Glucose is quickly absorbed directly into the blood. carbohydrates and simple sugar create a very high insulin Spike because of their quick absorption of sugar. This can explain the high amount of blood sugar after eating a meal that is full of carbohydrates.

Insulin is the key that opens the cell's door and helps nutrients and sugar to enter the cell. An excess amount of sugars will produce an excessive amount of insulin. An excess amount of insulin is produced to reduce the high levels of sugar in the blood. The high amount of sugar in the blood could potentially be dangerous to have for a very prolonged amount of time. I want you to think about insulin as à fan. When you enter a room and you turn on a fan for the first few minutes you will hear it and notice the sound that it makes pushing the air. After a little while, you will not hear it anymore. Your brain learned to ignore it and you forgot about it. Insulin is your body works in the same way. When you eat an excessive amount of sugar every single day, you will have a very high insulin spike every single day. After a while, your cells will learn that they do not need any more nutrients and sugars inside of them and they will stop reacting to insulin. This is what makes insulin resistance. Insulin resistance is what leads to high blood sugars in the blood. Your cells are not able to absorb the sugar that you have in your blood. This is what leads to high sugar blood levels and potentially prediabetes and type 2 diabetes.

It is very important to limit the number of carbohydrates that you consume on a regular basis. After you get insulin resistance your body needs to store the excess sugar somewhere. This sugar will be stored as fat. Primarily, this fat will be adipose tissue around your organs and liver creating a distended stomach. Your liver will store sugar as glycogen. Normally, your liver stores between 1700 and 2200 calories worth of sugar. When the liver is not able to store any more sugar, the excess sugar will be stored as fat around the liver. Creating a fatty liver can lead to cirrhosis and liver cancers. By limiting the amount of sugar you consume throughout the day can lead to the prevention of diabetes, obesity, fatty liver, and heart disease.

Many processed foods should be avoided at all costs. Many manufacturers create food that is highly palatable to the human taste buds. Highly processed foods are addictive. The taste that they have comes from the high amount of chemicals that they are made out of. Aside from all the carbohydrates, there are chemicals like MSG, maltodextrin, dextrin, aspartame, and many other chemicals. Manufacturers use chemicals to make food taste better than what it is. Many of these foods are made with low-quality oils. Oils like sunflower oil, safflower oil, soybean oil, and vegetable oil. These oils are very low quality and man-made, you need to avoid them at all cost. They have a high amount of omega-6 fatty acids. Omega-6 fatty acids are necessary, but an excess amount of them can create unnecessary inflammation inside and outside your body. You should always consume oils like extra virgin olive oil, coconut oil, avocado oil, and nut oils. These oils are high in omega-3 fatty acids. Omega-3 fatty acids are very beneficial for your health. Generally, we want to have more omega-3 fatty acids than omega-6 fatty acids. This will prevent inflammation in your body and have the added benefit of being very beneficial for your brain health. Your brain is made out of omega-3 fatty acids especially EPA and DHA found in Seafood.

Many processed foods are processed meats and pre-packaged meals. You should not eat them. Many of them are full of unnecessary carbohydrates, dangerous chemicals, and low-quality oils. My advice is to read the label of the food that you buy. You will notice many of the package foods contain multiple types of sugar. These sugars are corn syrup, honey, and agave nectar. These foods have many chemicals that are harmful and inflammatory Like MSG and artificial sweeteners. They also have low-quality oils like margarine and many other man-made oils. These ingredients that you do not know how to pronounce or you do not have in your kitchen should be avoided at all costs. Many of these ingredients are there to create an exotoxin response in your brain to make you addicted to them. It is good to avoid these chemicals and food and not take the risk of trusting a manufacturer with chemicals you might not know if they are good for you.

Many of these foods and chemicals are used to make you addicted to them. Many of these chemicals are like a drug to our body. When a person ingests a drug they might feel relaxed and happy. Your brain produces a hormone called dopamine. Dopamine is used for the feeling and sensation of happiness. Your brain loves dopamine. Every single time you take this drug the effect of dopamine is lower and lower. You can also think about the fan example, your brain learned to ignore dopamine. After a little while, your brain will start craving more and more all of the good feelings that dopamine produces. This is what creates an addiction. Many foods that are high in carbohydrates like desserts, potato, pasta, and bread make us feel good when we eat them. They produce the same dopamine response in your brain like a drug does. After we eat carbohydrates, an hour or two later we feel hungry again. We crave more of those tasty carbohydrates. Many chemicals like MSG have the same exotoxin effect in your body. Many restaurants like fast food and Chinese takeout use tons of MSG. Monosodium glutamate has a very similar effect on dopamine as sugar does. It will excite your brain, make you feel good and pleasant. After a little while, you feel hungry again because you'll start craving more and more of the same food because you want to feel happy again.

You might be wondering, what do I eat? carbohydrates are not bad to have in a balanced diet. You need to find carbohydrates in the form of nutrient-dense foods. An example of nutrient-dense foods is broccoli, spinach, cabbage, and kale. I consider these foods to be high-quality carbohydrates. You not only get sugar, but you also get vitamins and minerals like vitamin C, potassium, iron, and lots of antioxidants. You need to find the right daily amount of carbohydrates for you and your lifestyle. For me, 7 to 12 cups of vegetables every single day is my happy amount of high-quality carbohydrates. Allowing me the healthiest diet I can possibly find. Instead of processed meats, you can eat high-quality non-processed food and meats. Instead of buying hot dogs and frozen chicken patties. You can buy fresh chicken and fresh beef. You know these foods are only one ingredient and when you cook them you will know exactly what you put in it. You will not depend on a manufacturer to give you food and ingredients that may be harmful to you. Please do your best to buy foods that are 1 to 10 ingredients only. This will guarantee you that you will buy high quality instead of convenience or quantity. Look for foods like salmon, steak, sardines, and many other single-ingredient foods that are the highest quality you can afford. Do not buy the cheapest oil to cook with, buy oils like coconut oil, avocado oil, and olive oil. Avoid all processed oils like sunflower oil, cottonseed oil, and vegetable oil.

After a while of following these guidelines, you will find yourself looking for low carb, high quality minimally processed foods. Making the switch from low quality processed food to the best quality you can afford. This will make your life a better and healthier life by itself. It is not the only thing that you need to create a healthy living that you can be proud of. This is enough to get started. Please avoid high carbohydrate foods. Highly processed fast foods and convenience foods. Look for things that have 1 to 10 ingredients and make sure to avoid all of those foods that have chemicals to make them taste better than what they are.

CHAPTER III

MISTAKES TO AVOID

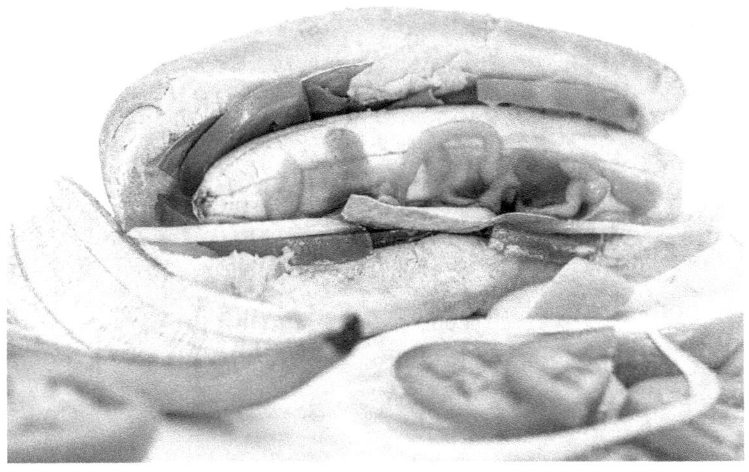

There are many mistakes that you need to know how to avoid, to have a successful healthy lifestyle. I have come across many people who have failed in their healthy lifestyle because of these simple mistakes anyone can avoid. I was one of the people that made similar mistakes and I learned from past experiences that they can be avoided and fixed. To have a healthy living you can be proud of, there are a couple of things that you can keep in mind about these mistakes. We have to make mistakes in our healthy lifestyle to grow and become a better us. Mistakes can lead to research and research can help us gain more knowledge about the topic that we're trying to learn about.

The first mistake that you need to be aware of is not reading the labels. labels in our food are there to help us make the healthiest choices for our life. Many manufacturers have found ways to trick us by using clever methods like portion sizes, different names for the same ingredients, and sketchy chemicals. The first thing you need to pay attention to is the portion size you want to make sure the item you're buying is an appropriate serving size. Sometimes we buy things that look healthy for us. We look at the item and sometimes look at the calories and think this item is great. We need to look at the serving size because the calories could only come from 1/2 of the whole item. I have seen as low as 1/8 of the item. This is why it is very important to check the serving size. We might think the healthiest item we just bought might be great for us but it's only a serving size of 1/8 per serving. If we eat the whole thing we might be in a huge calorie surplus. The second part about reading the label is different names for the same ingredient. You might think fructose corn syrup is different from corn syrup. It is the same thing. We have to keep in mind, many manufacturers are finding out that we are getting smarter about the food that we eat. They take advantage of the people that do not know how to read a label. They use words that mean the same thing but are written in a different way to confuse those buyers who are educated about labels. Many buyers don't see the word or the ingredient they might be trying to avoid and end up buying something they shouldn't. An example of this practice can be sugar, glucose, corn syrup, and many other syrups like molasses. They mean that the food item has sugar but it's to confuse you. When you go to the supermarket, please take your time to read the labels and the ingredients. If you have a phone with you, you can type the words that you see in the label. You can make sure it's safe to eat and what the word means does it mean. Don't be afraid to spend a little bit more time inside of a supermarket. You will end up making better choices. The third thing you need to look for in a label is the chemicals. Like I explained before in the chapter of quality there are many chemicals that can harm us. The first step when identifying dangerous chemicals is very simple: If you can pronounce the name or not. Many of the chemicals in food are written in chemical names. If you are a chemist you might know what they are and if they are harmful to you. If you are a person that has no knowledge about science or chemistry, you might find yourself stuck just by saying the name. Most likely if you do not know how to pronounce it, you do not know what it is or what it does. The second step to identify a dangerous chemical, it's to think or check if you have it in your kitchen. If you do not have it in your kitchen most likely you should not trust that chemical. By following these 2 easy steps you will avoid 90% of processed foods and frozen meals. Before I explain the second mistake you have to keep in mind some foods that are healthy for you may be written in the chemical name. One example of this can be vinegar. Vinegar is an acid that can be written by the name of acetic acid.

The second mistake I made at the beginning of my healthy Journey was not buying whole foods. I would buy pre-packaged or pre-made things that would be easier for me to cook. This is a huge mistake because many of these meals are full of preservatives to make them last longer on the shelves. Have you ever wondered if the food that you cook at home only lasts between one and two weeks in your refrigerator? Food in the store that looks similar to yours can be frozen for many months without going bad. These foods are full of many preservatives because 90% of grocery stores will lose money if they buy foods to sell to the public that can only last a couple of weeks. Many supermarkets are composed of many processed foods and items meant to make money off of you. One of the things I always explain to my clients is manufacturers do not care about your health. For example, broccoli is a whole food, broccoli is not adding any chemicals to itself to taste better than what it is for you. Broccoli does not have any intention to capitalize and make money from you. Manufacturers take this broccoli and process it with chemicals and preservatives to make it taste better and last longer. This makes many people buy processed broccoli. Manufacturers only care about money, they do not care about your health. This is why buying real food as broccoli and spinach will automatically improve your health. These whole food items are only one ingredient. There are no preservatives and no chemicals to worry about. When you buy whole food items you can season them any way you want. At the end of the day, you will know everything that you put in it and you know everything about it. There will be 0 MSG, 0 flavor enhancement, 0 preservatives. You will change your healthy lifestyle just by doing these simple steps. Looking for items that have simple ingredients and the least ingredients as possible. If you pick an item ingredients list that is a wall of text you should not read it, you should avoid it. The more ingredients that it has the more chemicals and processing that it is. By doing this you will not be putting your health in the hands of someone that does not care about your health. You will be putting your health in the hands of yourself. you will be responsible to keep yourself healthy and you'll be accountable for the things that you eat. Whole Foods would let you control your health that way you want to control it.

One of the biggest things that affected my progress while trying to build a healthy lifestyle was the lack of exercise. Exercise is the most powerful tool against stress, many health problems, and gaining weight. When I started my healthy lifestyle, I started walking everywhere. After a little while, I lost weight. This is when I started to run, running was the perfect exercise for me. I felt great after I did it and I felt accomplished because I did something productive. My mistake started to show when I started losing muscle. Long steady cardio it's great to keep you in shape but this exercise wasn't intense enough for me to keep my muscle. This is when I decided that I needed to lift weights. You need to find a balance between an exercise that will keep you in shape like cardio or swimming and an exercise that will keep you in the best intensity potential to be healthy like lifting weights or doing calisthenics. Not doing exercise early enough in my journey allowed me to go from one extreme of obesity to another extreme of being too skinny. You need to find an exercise that works for you. You can find love in any exercise as long as you move your body in a way that you enjoy it. Exercises could be yoga, CrossFit, or even powerlifting. Exercise can be your way to become healthy. All you need to keep in mind is every struggle that you get will help you become better. You will become the best version of yourself. Lifting weights and running is the perfect balance for me to stay lean and gain muscle the whole year. Look for exercises that will make you say to yourself "I am happy that I found this exercise and I feel so accomplished that I found it." Exercises can help with stress. Stress is a hormone produced by adrenal glands that is inversely related to insulin. It will stop insulin from working and opening the cell's door. High amounts of stress can cause high blood sugar levels and breakdown of muscle. This can lead to many diseases like type 2 diabetes. Sometimes many diabetics and pre-diabetics are very stressed people. If they calm down a little bit, their diabetes will become better. Later in this book, you learn what I do to control stress.

One of the mistakes I see many people do is not measuring your food. I am not asking you to measure your food forever. What you should do is measure your food until you feel comfortable knowing the portion sizes of all of the food that you eat. Food requirements and calories are different for every single person. You need to know and eat the appropriate calories that you need throughout your day. Eating below this calorie amount can help you lose weight. Do not attempt to eat super low calories in a day to lose weight. Calorie restriction diets do not work. Your body is an adaptable machine; it will adjust to everything that you throw at it. Eating a huge calorie deficit will lead to your body slowing down every single moment that you do, to have enough energy to live. Calorie restriction can lead you to feel tired and lethargic. Making you go back and binge food, making you gain all the weight you lost. By not restricting calories and only eating in a 5% to 10% calorie deficit or eating 200 to 350 fewer calories per day. Will lead you to a sustainable weight loss in the long-term. Measuring your food will allow you to know how much food you need in a day and how much less you can eat to lose weight. By a month or two of measuring your food, you will know the amount of food you need to be healthy enough to stay in shape and strong enough to look great.

By avoiding these mistakes and correcting them you will most likely have a successful lifestyle and healthy living that you can be proud of. By starting to look for quality, avoiding to eat processed foods, reading labels, doing exercise, and measuring your food, you will find a way to live a healthy life and think about your health first. You will put your health in your own hands to find a way that will work for you.

CHAPTER IV

FIND SUPPORT

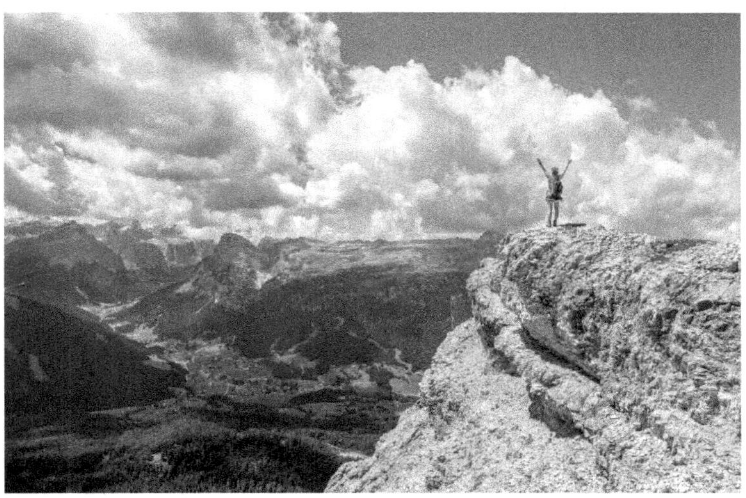

To be the healthiest person you can be, sometimes there's difficulties and plateaus that will discourage you from going forward. It's important to acknowledge that every single day we see thousands of people throughout our day. Every single relationship and interaction with other people it's an opportunity for you to grow as a person. In this chapter, you will learn how to create a robust relationship and Network. Throughout my journey, I realized I would have never done it if I was alone. Many people that supported me, inspired me to keep going.

The first thing that I always tell people, throughout their journey, is that there will be many people that will not support you and try to tell you that you cannot make it. It is important to find four to five people who are honest, reliable, and truthful to the words. These people have different purposes in your life and will help you achieve your goals easier. These people will not only help you in your healthy living but also help you in your career and other aspects of your life. Support Is a powerful tool that you can use as motivation inside of your journey and it will help you to stay accountable to yourself and to the people that believe in you.

We'll start by looking for people that will support you no matter what you choose to do. The support you need for your healthy living can be described as a house. You need a person to be your foundation, another person to be the pillars, another person to be the walls, and another person to be the roof. Your foundation should be someone that is ahead of you in life and you perceive this person as a role model. Your Foundation will help you to grow in your goals and help you grow in a network that you can use to grow yourself. An example of a role model could be a professor that I had in college. She allowed me to do research for her. The research experience and advice I got from this person allowed me to do research with other people and let me grow in a network of scientists and science figures. This made me become a well-known figure in the science community. Your foundation should be a person that is willing to Mentor you and make you grow in a network in the community that you're trying to grow in. A mentor for a healthy living could be a coach, nutritionist, or anyone who is ahead of you in the nutrition and fitness field. The second person that you need is a pillar. Pillars are used for support. This person is someone who's always there for you. They will ask about your life and support you in everything that you do. Your pillar is someone truthful and honest, someone, who is able to be upfront with you and tell you things that you are doing wrong. They will point out the mistakes that you're making. Also, this person will allow you to go forward in life in anything that you are willing to achieve. An example of this person could be friends that are always there for you and always ask you how are you doing and what are you doing. When this person sees that I'm doing something wrong or doing something that I shouldn't, they should let me know what I am doing wrong. Your person in your healthy living that you're trying to find does not have to be an expert in nutrition. It should be someone to tell you that you can do it. The third person that you need, the person that you need, is your walls. This person is able to do the same thing as support does and is able to do a little more. These people will take time off their day to spend it with you. This person is also honest and truthful to everything that they tell you. This person is what I call a best friend. They will support you no matter what and spend time with you no matter what. An example of a best friend can be someone who is willing and able to take time from the day to spend it with you. They will help you achieve your goals and dreams. This person is appreciative of everything you do and is willing and able to help you achieve everything that you want to do. Your best friend can be someone that is close to you and is already your best friend to make sure they become that bearing wall in your life. After this person, all you need is a roof. This person will help you achieve your goals in an easier way. This person will accompany you throughout your goal and throughout your healthy living that you can be proud of. This person will be there to do your healthy journey with you. This person will hold you accountable for your success in your goal. This person is counting on you to make it so they can make it. You can call this person a business partner. This can be anyone who's also looking to have a healthier lifestyle and has decided to help you and accompany you on your journey. This will give you the feeling that you're not doing this around or by yourself helping you achieve your goals easier and more successfully you won't do it alone.

You might be wondering, Where do I find these people? The first thing you have to do is write down ideal support. I called his ideal support your board of leaders. You will describe every single person from your mentor role model to your roof business partner. These people should have the characteristics of being honest and truthful. They should be able to support you with any goal that you want to achieve. They should be there for you to guide you and mentor you throughout your healthy living. An example of this description would be a person who is honest, this person will help me achieve my goals in my healthy Journey. This person cannot be someone that discourages me or says negative comments about my dreams. You can have a deadline by which you find these people. you can have as many people as you want. I have seen many boards of leaders who are only made of one, two people, and ten people.

Sometimes it might look like people don't want to support you. This is simply not true if you are honest about it and you are open to how many people know what you are doing in your life. They will be more than happy to support you. At the beginning of my business, I was embarrassed to tell anyone about it when I started to lose my fear of posting on social media and branding myself as someone of authority and people started supporting me. There were people that I never thought would help me throughout my journey. People only encourage me and share and encourage me and share my content so other people could support me too. Sometimes all we need to do is to ask for it. It might be difficult at first but you have to lose your fear, lose your fear, and become an authority within your group and many people will support you.

I am happy to say that I am your support. I want you to succeed in your healthy living and anything you are trying to ask in life. I am very confident you will achieve your goals and your fitness journey. Soon in this book, I will show you how to write a goal and how you can find your successful board of leaders. Your goals can be written for anything that you want to achieve in life. Even though this book is aimed to help you throughout your healthy journey. You can use this book in any situation or any goal and achievement you want to accomplish. Your board of leaders is the support that you need to help you get where you want to go. After a while, you will notice that more and more people will join you and support you. You will feel inspired by them. You will be held accountable by many people that want you to succeed. Many of these people are waiting for you to make it so they can feel inspired to Make it.

By looking for people that will inspire you to become better. You will most likely find it easier to succeed in your

Healthy Living that you can be proud of. Many people who do not think support can be helpful for them or how to support will Inspire them. When I started running, I used to go to a track that was full of professional athletes. They were very quick around the track. They were training to be the fastest at a 400-meter dash. When I was in the middle of my journey and stuck not getting any faster. The coach from the professional running team came to me after a hard day trying to get better and told me "good job young man" These little words of support made me want to become better. They filled me with motivation to keep going. You will catch the attention of people who are ahead of you in the journey and are able and willing to help you. After this moment of motivation, I trained my body to run for long distances for a long amount of time. I realized I was good at running for three to four miles every single run that I did. If I never heard motivation from some people ahead of me, and not had any people supporting me and people doing it with me, I most likely would have failed.

CHAPTER V

HEALTH BENEFITS

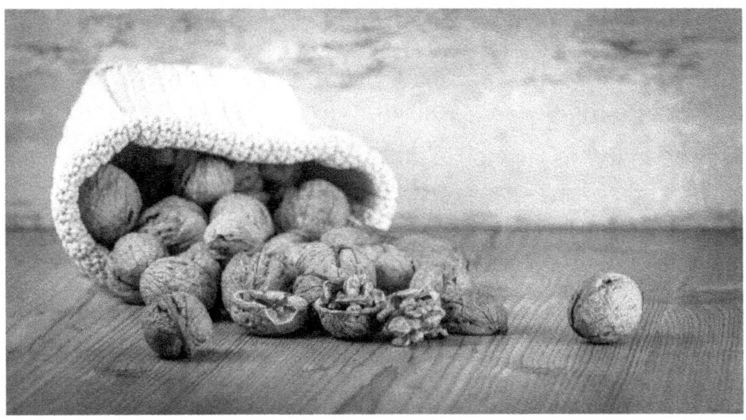

Right now, I would like to speak to you about the health benefits of a healthy whole food diet so you can have. how many people believe diseases are being caused by genetic inheritance. These people are not wrong, Many people are predisposed to having illnesses easier than others. Diet plays a big role in diseases you may or may not have. In this chapter, you will learn about the diseases caused by eating habits that can be changed and avoided at costs.

One of these diseases is type 2 diabetes. Many people think fat is the enemy when the real enemy is sugar. Sugar will trigger insulin more than any other thing we consume. The more sugar we eat the more insulin for your body will produce. Insulin is like the storage hormone. Everything that you eat needs to go inside the cells. Insulin is the key that opens the door for nutrients to flow in. We know insulin is necessary for you to be alive. Every food that we eat has an insulin response. Some foods will have a higher response to insulin than others. Overconsumption of sugar will have a higher insulin response. Forcing your pancreas to work extra hard. After a long period of time, you consumed an abundance of sugar. The high amount of sugar will cause your body to stop responding to insulin. The poor response is known as insulin resistance. High amounts of insulin resistance inside your body lead to excess sugar in the blood. Your cells do not want any more sugar inside of them. They shut the door against insulin and this is what causes diabetes. The problem with having high sugar consumption would be gaining weight. The high amount of sugar makes it very dangerous to have in the blood.

I believe it is a very good thing to lower stress. I will give you a couple of steps on how to manage stress. The first thing I do to manage stress it's just to breathe. Breathing is a very powerful tool for your health and your life. When you are in a stressful situation all you have to do is breathe. Breathe in slowly and breathe out twice as slow. For example, when I feel stressed, I breathe in for 3 seconds then I breathe out for 6 seconds. Why do I do this? Believe it or not, when you breathe in, your heart rate increases, and when you breathe out, your heart rate decreases. The longer that you breathe in, then the twice as long that you breathe out. The slowdown of your heart rate will calm you. This happens because your body is not releasing cortisol. This is why it is very important for you to breathe in slowly and breathe out slowly. You become calmer and this will release stress drastically. Stress it's a hormone in your body we call it cortisol. Cortisol is a type of steroid hormone that is produced by the adrenal glands. It is related to insulin, we can think about cortisol as an extra door in the cell against insulin. Cortisol will stop insulin from storing nutrients and sugar inside of the cells. This will lead you to have an increase in insulin resistance in your body. Creating more high blood sugar problems and promoting diabetes. Many diabetics and pre-diabetics are just really stressed people. To lower the amount of cortisol in your body is to breathe. Remember, when you breathe in, do it slowly when you breathe out, do it twice as slow. This will promote insulin sensitivity and reduce the risk of type 2 diabetes. One thing that you need to know about cortisol, it is necessary to have cortisol in our body for regulating blood pressure and blood sugar levels. We need to have a specific amount of cortisol in our body to regulate many body functions. An excess amount will lead to constricted blood vessels, produce high blood sugars, and high blood pressure. We have to understand that our body is regulated by many hormones and minerals that need to be in balance.

Healthy fats are Omega-3 fatty acids. Eating more omega-3 fatty acids will make your body have less inflammation. You have to be careful with omega-6 fatty acids; they are more common on low-quality food. Let me make this clear, you do need omega-6 fatty acids. The problem begins with eating an abundance of omega-6. Your body will be thrown off balance between your omega-3 and omega-6 fatty acids. It will make you more inflamed and lead to things like bloating, high blood pressure, and some types of cancer. The problem with having high sugar consumption would be gaining weight. The high amount of sugar makes it very dangerous to have in the blood. For example, fast-food restaurants have foods made out of wheat in the form of refined carbohydrates and meat that is the lowest quality. This processed food contains a high amount of omega-6 fatty acids and sugar that causes a big insulin spike. This will make many nutrients and sugars get into the cell. Once the cell is full, the excess will be stored as fat. It is important to limit the number of carbohydrates you eat. Many healthy foods will not have enough sugar to cause a high enough insulin Spike. An excess of carbohydrates in our food will cause an excess of fat. Sugars and poor quality food leads to high inflammation, clogged arteries, and heart disease. Blame sugars, not the fats. Your brain is mostly made out of fat. Especially the fat found in seafood which is an omega-3 fatty acid (EPA and DHA). Having a moderate fat and moderate protein every single day along with the low amount of carbs is beneficial.

Some organs like your heart are required to use sugar, but you should not be worried about having an absence of sugar in your body. Your body has the ability to make carbohydrates out of protein and fat whenever your body needs it. By eating enough protein your body would use the excess proteins to produce carbohydrates by the process of gluconeogenesis. In the process of gluconeogenesis, your body will take protein and process it to create the sugar that is needed for your body to function. Something important for you to remember, your body only needs about a teaspoon of sugar through your bloodstream. A teaspoon is 4 to 5 grams. There should always be only 4 to 5 grams of carbohydrates circulating through our blood system. The excess sugar will be stored as fat as a way of your body to protect you. It's a way for your body to store energy safely for a rainy day and utilize it through the process of ketosis.

Fatty cuts of meat are quickly becoming more popular as many people discover a healthy diet. One tablespoon of olive oil into your salad and cooking in a little bit of butter is everything that you need for a successful healthy diet. A healthy diet is not a diet to eat poor quality food. I take advantage of this to have a better quality of eating. It's a way of me eating more salad and eating better quality meats. As I progress and discover new things that would help me achieve my goal in health and fitness. I have found that a healthy diet is so much easier to stay fit for the whole year. The lack of carbohydrates make me stay lean, my body doesn't have to hold so much water or make me bloated. High-quality food makes my body work more efficiently at preventing many diseases by boosting my immune system. My body doesn't have to deal with all of the inflammation caused by low quality processed foods.

Many cancer cells are broken. Their machinery to adapt has changed. That allows them to reproduce without control. This uncontrolled reproduction made the cell lose its machine adaptability. This means cancer cells cannot adapt to fat burning. This leads to many cancer cells starving until they die. Cancer cells are only able to use sugar for fuel. When your sugar is low, your body will prioritize the usage of sugar with organs that are needed the most. Organs like your brain and your heart will use the sugar first before any cell on your body. These organs are more essential for your body to survive, cancer cells need to have a surplus of sugar to be able to thrive. Low sugar will lead them to have a shortage of food inhibiting the growth and leading to their death.

CHAPTER VI

HAVE A GOAL

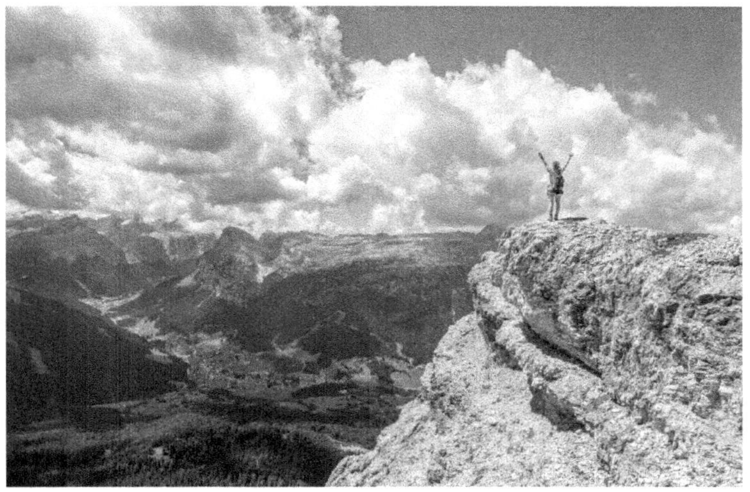

Many people have asked me How to stay consistent with such a strict diet. My answer is by having a lot of desire. Desire is the ability to want to achieve your goals no matter the situation. Desire makes you not only want to improve but deciding to become an improvement. For example, if you want to be rich you don't say "I want money" or "I want to be rich". You will tell yourself "I will be rich". A goal has to be specific and have a motivation and a strong desire to 50 achieve it. When I started my weight-loss journey, I said to myself, "in the next 6 months, I am going to lose at least 100 pounds. I will lose this 100 pounds by eating the best quality of food and by having the best exercise routine to help me burn all the extra fat in my body."

Please take a piece of paper and write down your goals. You want your goals to be what you want to achieve, and why. Read it out loud to yourself every single morning and every single night. The repetition of this goal will make you believe it. Your faith and desire for this goal will become stronger the more you repeat it. The more that you repeat this goal to yourself, the more often that you will have this goal in mind. Over time, You will keep your goal in mind and you will start looking for ways to achieve it in your daily life. You will become better at what you're trying to achieve

The things that you believe are the things that you will attract. If you believe that your business will do well, you will attract money. If you believe you can gain muscle and stay fit the whole year, you will attract what you believe. Have the desire for the things that you want to achieve in life. Make a specific goal that will make you believe your set goal until you become it. At first, you might think it is impossible to make it happen. Over weeks and months of believing and having the desire to do it. You will have your goal in your hands.

Another thing that will help you achieve your goals and anything that you want to do in life. It's by having faith. There is no way that you can feel the desire if you don't have faith. You are what you desire. If you do not have faith it will be difficult to become the person that you want to be. I am where I want to be today because my faith is so strong, I have the desire to achieve my goals. In this set amount of goals, I gave myself the ability to think that every goal is possible at all costs.

I encourage everyone to take their time and map out where they want to go. Read that goal over and over and always seek for the things that will help you achieve that goal. There is no reason and no excuse to let go and fail. All you have to do is review your goal every single day. Keep it in mind until you believe it. You'll become your dream. Right now my goal is to become more muscular and be more fit. I tell myself every day the steps and things that I want to achieve.

A big reason to not be around a person that will not let you achieve your goals is that they will affect your mindset. It would not be the best idea to be around a person or a group of people that think in a negative way about you. For example, I had a group of friends when I started thinking about being a better person and started my weight-loss journey. These people told me that I could not do it. They told me that I was lazy, fat, and clumsy. I had a strong desire and faith that I could do it. I stopped being around negative people that will discourage me. I found a group of people that would support me and help me become a better person. You should limit the amount of time you spend with people that will discourage you from becoming a better you. If a person or group of people tell you that your goals are impossible, you tell them that you will make it happen no matter what it takes. You will replace these people with people that have the same mindset as you. Find growth-oriented people to help you grow as a person.

Also, you want to stay away from the people that enable you to do the opposite of what you're trying to achieve.

After your goal is written, all you have to do is take action and look for people that will support you and your goal. This will help you become a better you. Always have your goal in mind and look for things that help you achieve your goals. If you see a business opportunity, take it. If you find something to help yourself, do it. It's worth being healthy no matter what the situation is. Make Health your first priority.

Remember, the goals have to be very specific. They need a specific what, specific how, specific deadline, and specifically why. These steps will help you map out the specific steps that you need to take to accomplish your goal. To make these goals successful, you need to have this goal in a place that you can see it. Remind yourself to read it every morning and every night. The repetition of this goal will make it easier for you to remember it. Over time your mind will create a radar that will help you identify the little things in life that will allow you to accomplish your goal. You will repeat your goal to yourself so much that you will believe it to the point that you will become it.

You have the confidence to become what you want to be. What you want to call yourself, whatever you call yourself it's whatever you already are. Have the faith and the discipline combined with a desire to do the things, that make you happy. Find people to support you. People that believe in you when nobody does. When someone believes in you, you can believe in yourself. If someone that is not part of your body knows that you can make it very far. You should believe in yourself. You should believe you can make it. I believe in you, I know you can achieve great things in your life.

CHAPTER VII

EXERCISE

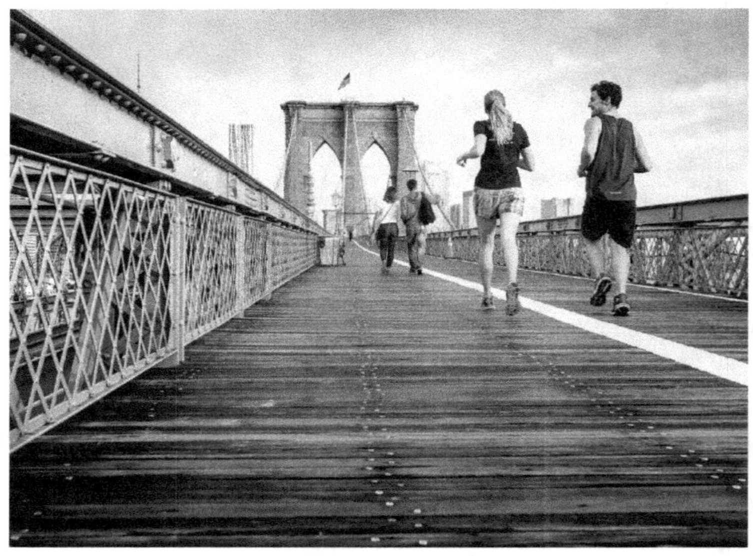

Lifestyle is nothing without exercise, it's like having food without a pair of chopsticks. You need to do at least some form of exercise that will allow you to feel great after you are finished. Exercise is very important for our wellbeing.

Exercise is very powerful for lowering stress and making you feel better.

It's important to have a good workout routine that will make you push yourself enough to see change but not too intense to hurt yourself. I should have done this from the beginning and started working out in a gym. Right now, I go to the gym and perform a workout that is challenging enough to see my body change but not too hard to hurt my body. Running helps me burn the surplus of calories that I consume. This helps me stay in shape. You do not have to do this. The first thing that you need is a healthy balanced diet, the second thing is the desire and faith to keep going, and the third thing is to find a way to move your body in a way that you enjoy it. Examples could be, walking, running, and swimming. You can do anything as long as you do some exercise and eat good quality foods.

Before I started my journey I found my root cause to be the lack of exercise and a lack of healthy habits. Before I changed something, I looked for the best exercises for me to do and the types of healthy habits I needed to do. When we do exercise we feel great because we release dopamine to our body. This is what makes you feel relaxed, happy, and gives us the feeling we accomplished something. Doing exercise helped my body become healthy especially in the cardiovascular system.. You need to find a lifestyle that will help you exercise away all of the things that make you stressed. You need to find a way to keep learning and keep understanding things.

The right exercise that works for you is an amazing discovery for your life. You need to try as many different types of exercise that you can think of. If you think yoga is good for you, try it. If you think CrossFit will be good for you, try it. You need to stay consistent. If you choose yoga, give it at least 3 months to decide if you're good at it or not. Everyone at the beginning of something sucked. In the beginning, when I started running, I could not run for 3 miles. I could not run for 30 minutes straight but now I can. I can put on my running shoes and just run.

Sometimes having a large amount of something low quality will end up hurting you more than helping you. If I have never gone down to the gym and started lifting weights, I probably would have been too skinny from losing weight. I learned so much in a gym I am able to do the same exercises by using my own body weight. This is why consistency quality and learning is so important. When I say "you got this" and "you can" is because I believe in you. I myself was able to find a better quality of life through a healthy diet, running, and exercise. I was able to think about my health first. Everything that I do around my life is about health and how I can become healthier.

If you start bodybuilding and you have a goal to body build you need to start calling yourself a bodybuilder. When I started I didn't want to call myself a runner or an athlete. Exercise will make you become an athlete. It's up to you to call yourself an athlete, or a runner, or a bodybuilder. It's up to you if you want to become a better version of yourself. You will not be a beginner bodybuilder forever or a beginner runner forever. You want to learn something that will take you from being a beginner to an advanced level. You can do it all you need is to have confidence in yourself.

Exercise will help you keep stress low. It will help you stay in your ideal weight and you make you feel accomplished at the end. Find an exercise that will make you move your body in a way that you enjoy it. Look for ways that will help you live longer. Exercise will teach you to become better. The skills you learn doing exercise will carry over to other aspects of your life.

The best exercises that you can do in a healthy lifestyle are cardio, walking, and aerobic exercise. Long steady cardio is optimal for burning a lot of calories. Many people think going to the gym and lifting heavy weights would be a great exercise to burn fat. This is not true because you're making a maximum effort for a short time. Having short outbreaks of powerful moves will lead you to burn calories but it will not be sustainable to burn a lot of calories for a very long time. Long steady cardio is great to burn a lot of calories because you will be running for long distances for a very long time. Where the intensity is not hard enough to make you stop but not easy enough to burn fewer calories. Long steady cardio works because you will deplete your glycogen storage after the first 15 minutes of running. After this glycogen is depleted you will start burning your own fat from your body. The same thing can be said about walking. Walking is a low intensity, low impact exercise that allows you to do it for long periods of time without causing any extra stress on the body. Doing these exercises and staying active will be the perfect recipe to create healthy living. Doing low impact exercises for long periods of time is a perfect recipe to burn fat and reduce stress in your body. Aerobics exercises are exercises you're able to while breathing and speaking full sentences without any problem. I always advise anyone to stay active and move their body at least once a day every day. This will help them keep a very healthy lifestyle avoiding all of the diseases and risks associated with low movement. For example, you can take the stairs instead of the electric stairs or the elevator. You can walk the longest route to your home and take very long walks around relaxing places. After a while, you will be able to run and stay active no matter what you choose to do in life.

SUBSCRIBE TO MY NEWSLETTER

WWW.NEYFIDELROSARIO.COM

READ MY OTHER BOOK:

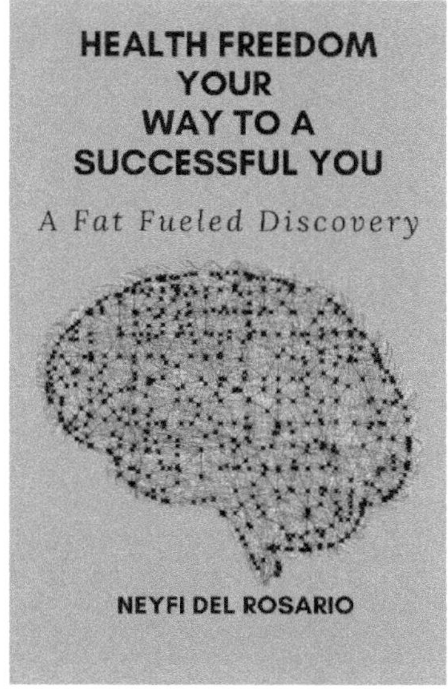

www.ingramcontent.com/pod-product-compliance
Lightning Source LLC
Chambersburg PA
CBHW050658250726
48662CB00002B/743